Own Movember

How to Grow More Facial Hair, Feel Manlier, and Overcome Your Genetics

By Thurman Darby

PUBLISHED BY MUNSON MEDIA
Copyright © 2014 Thurman Darby

All Rights Reserved. This book or any portion thereof may not be reproduced or used in any manner whatsoever without the express written permission of the publisher except for the use of brief quotations in a book review.

ISBN: 978-1511869324

Cover Image © Sfio Cracho / Shutterstock.com
Inside Image © Alexander Potapov / Shutterstock.com

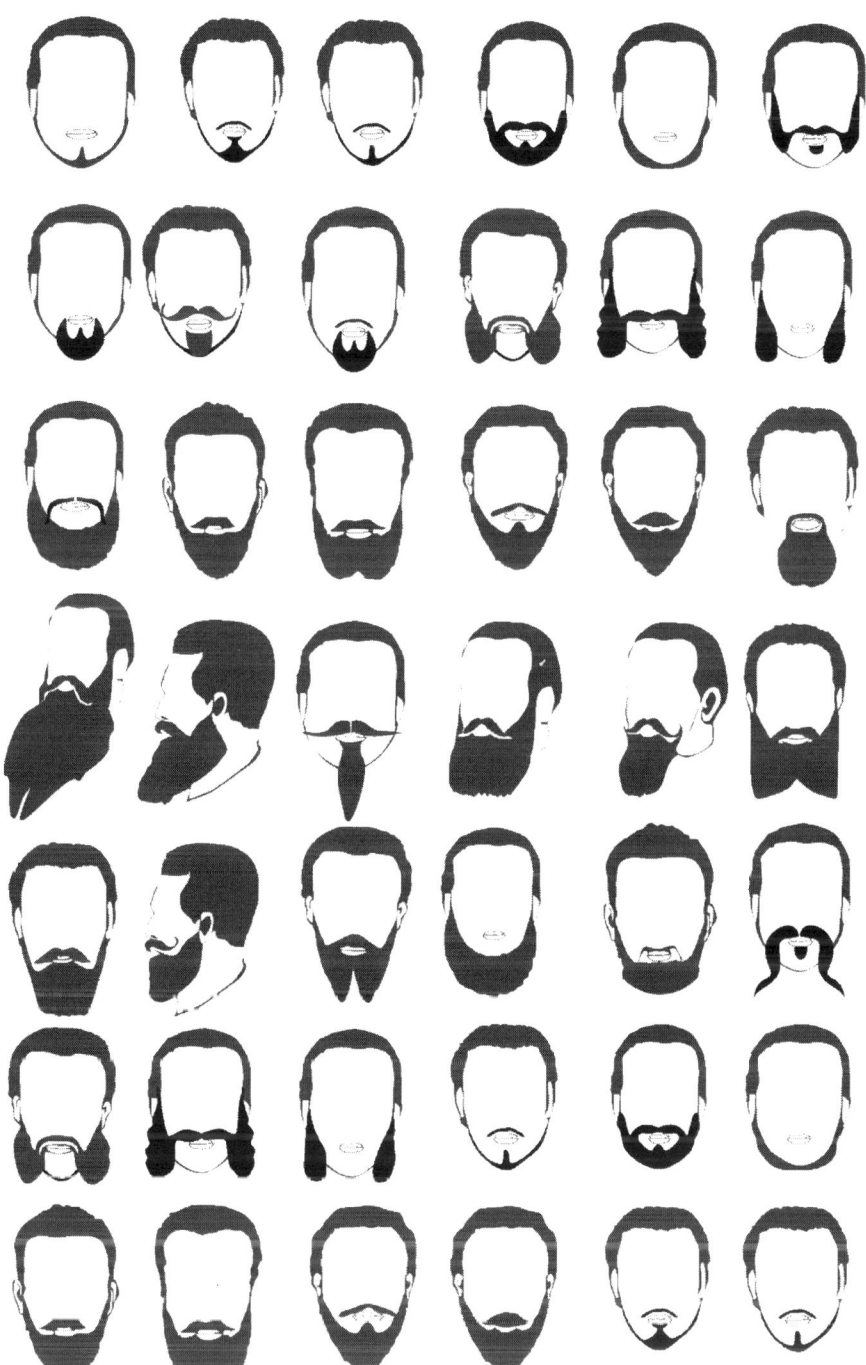

Thurman Darby

Disclaimer

There is not a "Dr." in front of my name or an "M.D." at the end of it. I am not a doctor, although sometimes I play one on Halloween. Please do not pursue any of the advice presented in this book without properly assessing whether it is safe for you under the guidance of a doctor.

Contents

1 Why Beards Rule

2 Baboons to Baby Faces: Explaining Differences in Facial Hair Among Men

3 Removing Beard Barriers

4 Cross Your T's: The Importance of Testosterone

5 The Method Behind Our Madness

6 Beard Food

7 The Bigger Beard Workout

8 Testosterone Therapy

9 Rogaine: What Works on Your Head Should Work on Your Face, Right?

10 Household Recipes

11 Let's Get Surgical

12 Growing, Coloring, Maintaining

13 Odds and Ends

Final Words

Thurman Darby

Preface

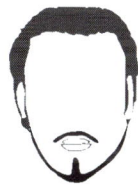 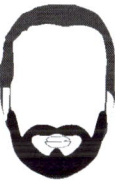 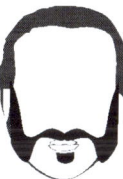

Things have never been worse for the "boy face"—the unfortunate souls unable to grow adequate facial hair. Facial hair has long been associated with wisdom, virility, and above all, manliness. A full beard is one of the clearest indications of healthy testosterone levels in the body; which is wired into men's and women's brains to be a highly desirable trait.

The swinging pendulum of popular style has also swung against the boy face—billboards, magazines, and televisions are covered with perfectly stubbled and bearded faces—without a doubt, facial hair is in!

If that isn't bad enough, every November has become an annual reminder of the boy face's ineptitude. "Movember"—the fantastic annual event where men grow moustaches to raise money for men's health issues—has grown from local fundraiser to worldwide phenomenon in less than a decade. Unfortunately, a quirky and clever way to bring about much needed attention to men's health has transformed into an annual referendum on manliness. During Movember, the boy face gets chastised for being uncharitable at best and unmanly at worst.

I had been suffering from boy face my entire life. Everyone always said: "Be patient, it will grow in when you get older." I was in my thirties and had the facial hair coverage of Arizona desert foliage. My beard was best described as a sparse collection of whiskers complemented by charming patches of peach fuzz. It was horrible.

I had heard a million times from doctors that facial hair is dictated by genetics and that it was pointless to try and fight my genes. I was told I should be thankful that I didn't have to shave every day! Well, I wasn't willing to accept those answers or my genetic facial follicle growing deficiencies. There had to be a way to overcome my genetics and to turn the odds in my favour. I knew I was never going to be confused for a member of ZZ Top or Duck Dynasty, but I desperately wanted to grow a real beard. The date was November 30, 2013; I vowed that the following year's November would be different. I wouldn't just participate in the following year's Movember, I would own it!

This book lays out how I was able to go from Movember chump to champ. I'll give you some background as to why some men are able to grow a beard by lunch and why some can only manage a few whiskers. I'll discuss the latest research showing not only what facial hair projects to other men (and the opposite sex), but how it affects a man's perception of himself. Then I'll get to the good stuff. I'll discuss all the methods proven to help men grow more facial hair. This includes what I used (and didn't use) to dramatically increase my facial hair growth in less than a year.

I can't guarantee you anything. Your genetics dictate a lot of what grows (or doesn't grow) on your face. But there are absolutely ways to maximize and enhance what you currently have; I am living proof. A lot of the methods I discovered that improve a man's facial hair also improve his vitality and overall health and that is no coincidence. My whole life prior to November 2013 was spent being lazy, fat, and unhealthy. With the motivation I had to Own Movember, I was able to get into incredible shape and completely transform my life. Hopefully this book will inspire you to do the same.

Part I: Setting the Stage for Growth

1
Why Beards Rule

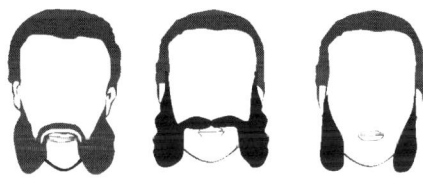

Facial hair profoundly influences how a man is judged by other people and the judgments he makes about himself. Let's start with the first one. Several academic studies have shown that men with beards are judged to be more masculine, dominant, self-confident, courageous, sincere, generous, industrious, and yes—attractive. A 2013 study published in the Journal of Evolution and Human Behavior looked at the perceived attractiveness of men with varying amounts of facial hair. Men sporting heavy stubble—defined as 10 days of growth without shaving—were rated most attractive by women compared to men with full beards, light stubble and clean-shaven looks.

The same study showed that women judged men with heavy stubble or full beards to be more masculine, healthier, and even have better parenting skills! The men in the study came to similar conclusions. Men found the full bearded gentlemen to be the most attractive, most healthy, most masculine, and also have the best parenting skills.

Another interesting finding was that men with light stubble—defined as five days of growth without shaving—were rated the worst across the board, even worse than the clean shaven men. This told me a few things: first, that five days growth is the "homeless man" look. It makes sense that a lot of men choose to begin growing a beard over an extended vacation from work to get past the light stubble phase. Second, there's clearly a threshold of facial hair coverage and thickness to be crossed before a beard becomes an attractive signal; peach fuzz patches are not going to cut it!

Sporting quality facial hair can definitely put your best face out to the world—but how does it make you feel about yourself? Turns out it changes your behavior and self-perception—even when the facial hair is fake! There hasn't been a lot of research done about this topic, but I found one study which had clean-shaven men self-evaluate while wearing either fake beards, bandanas, or nothing at all. The bearded group rated themselves as much more masculine than the other two groups, even though they knew the beards were fake—just seeing the outline of hair on their faces made them think of themselves as more manly. Self-perception affects behavior. If your brain is telling you that you're "manly", then you're more likely to act in an assertive and dominant manner than if your brain isn't receiving that signal.

So it's clear that facial hair is awesome, but why are there such differences in men's abilities to grow it? What separates the baboons from the baby faces?

2

Baboons to Baby Faces: Explaining Differences in Facial Hair Among Men

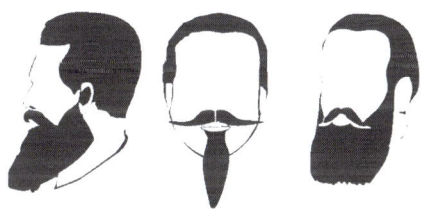

Men and women both have facial hair; it's true, and I'm not just talking about my great aunt Lorna. Beginning when we're in diapers, men's and women's faces and bodies get covered in vellus hair, or what's commonly referred to as "peach fuzz". The amount of vellus hair you have is determined by your genetics. Vellus hair is useless for our purposes until puberty—that's when androgens like testosterone run wild through a boy's body like the Cháng Jiāng River.

The androgens—which are a group of steroid hormones—bind to a boy's facial hair follicles and transform his peach fuzz into thicker, darker, "terminal" hair. The androgen/facial hair relationship is not nearly as strong after puberty but it definitely still applies. More androgens circulating around in a man's body means there's more of it available to bind to his hair follicles—which give more instructions to make his vellus hair thicker and darker. So case closed; low testosterone explains your boy face and you should start supplementing it immediately...is it really that simple?

I have an Italian friend—let's call him Vinny—who is obese, lazy, has the muscle tone of a watermelon, and is barely strong enough to lift a Venti coffee from Starbucks (he's single ladies if you're interested). Despite these shortcomings, he has one of the thickest beards known to man; his beard follicles have follicles! Another friend of mine—let's call him Tom—looks like he was chiseled out of stone and can lift a full beer keg over his head (I hate when he does that, the beer gets all foamy). Tom has decent facial hair coverage but cannot grow anything like Vinny. Now I'm not a doctor but I am a gambler, and I would bet a sizeable chunk of change that Tom has a higher testosterone level than Vinny.

That completely unnecessary paragraph is meant to dispel the biggest myth when it comes to beards—that men able to grow awesome beards have higher testosterone than men unable to grow much of anything. In fact, a large proportion of adult men have pretty similar levels of testosterone. There's clearly something else going on to explain the vast differences in men's facial hair growing abilities.

If a lot of men have about the same level of testosterone telling their facial hair to grow thicker and darker, then differences in facial hair must come down to how well their follicles listen to testosterone's instructions. Genetics are largely responsible for dictating how your facial hair responds to the presence of androgens. Some men's facial hair barely respond at all, while other men's are incredibly sensitive; it's the genetic lottery at work but it's not all bad news for the boy faces.

High androgen sensitivity with regards to facial hair often translates to the hair on a man's head. The problem is that scalp follicles react to androgens in a completely different way. Scalp follicles that are highly sensitive to androgens like Dihydrotestosterone (DHT) will shrink and cause the hair to fall out—so it's not all rainbows and lollypops for our baboon-faced friends!

Raising your androgen levels from your current baseline will vary in its effectiveness but it will almost certainly help your facial hair growing cause. One thing is 100 percent sure; if you are testosterone deficient, you will not be able to own Movember. In fact, there's a good chance the facial hair you do have will fall out! More on testosterone later, but for now let's address other "beard barriers" that you'll need to remove before you can Own Movember.

3
Removing Beard Barriers

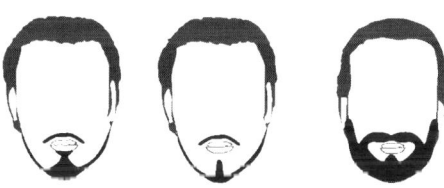

Before investing time and money in your beard growing skills, it's important to remove significant "beard barriers" that will undermine your efforts. Here are 4 important barriers to address immediately.

1. Get Enough Sleep

When you are asleep, your body regenerates and grows. Like actually—that's the time your body releases a significant amount of growth hormone. Also, most testosterone is made during deep REM (Rapid Eye Movement) sleep. A poor sleep cycle with less time spent in REM has been associated with low testosterone levels. Getting at least 6 hours of uninterrupted sleep is essential but try and to get as close to 8 hours as possible. Sleep deprivation is one of the most common factors associated with hair loss and according to a study published in the Journal of the American Medical Association, men sleeping 5 or fewer hours a night experienced a 15 percent drop in testosterone.

Own Movember Tip #1: Try to get at least 6 hours of uninterrupted sleep per night and preferably 8 hours total.

2. Manage Your Stress Levels

Stress causes all kinds of wear and tear on your body. It particularly attacks your immune system, which stunts your hair growth. It also increases production of cortisol, which lowers testosterone production. I know, I hate getting the "don't be stressed out" advice—thanks tips! Life is stressful; stress comes at us from all angles on a daily basis. Although a lot of the stress being inflicted on our lives is uncontrollable, how you manage it *is* controllable.

There's a saying that hair reveals stress. I had poorly managed my stress levels my entire life and it showed! I knew I would never Own Movember if my existing stress management continued. I took control of my stress by exercising more and I even began meditating and doing yoga regularly. I felt really silly doing the latter 2 but I have to tell you they do wonders. After a few weeks of yoga, I noticed myself becoming more insulated to daily stressors and I had significantly more energy. Yoga also boosts circulation which is great for hair growth.

Own Movember Tip #2: Working out, yoga, and mediation are the best and easiest natural stress insulators.

3. Lay off the Cigs

As if you needed another reason! The nicotine from cigarette smoke affects your body's ability to absorb nutrients needed for proper hair growth. Smoking also negatively affects your blood pressure and circulation. Oh and it kills you.

Own Movember Tip #3: Lay off the cigs, man!

4. Take Care of Your Skin

When your hair follicles are blocked with grime or dirt, hair cannot grow. It's crucial to keep your face clean to allow your hair follicles to sprout up properly. Ensure to wash your face twice a day or any time it's dirty with sweat or oil. Be careful not to over wash or use harsh products as these will dry your face out and block your pores with dead skin cells. Use a moisturizer to help with this issue and to keep your skin in top form. This was a very important realization for me as I have very dry skin. I also exfoliate my face once a week with an exfoliator with eucalyptus. It feels great on my skin and the eucalyptus helps stimulate hair growth.

Own Movember Tip #4: Wash your face and moisturize twice a day to keep your pores and hair follicles clean. Hair will not grow properly if your pores are blocked.

4

Cross Your T's: The Importance of Testosterone

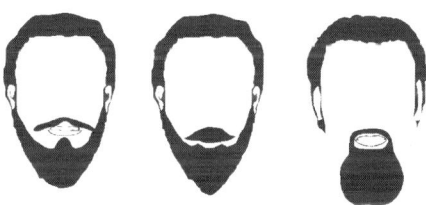

Testosterone is the essence of masculinity. Everything that defines what makes a man a man is transformed by this hormone. It's the fuel for all male characteristics and affects our mood, energy, sexual desire, muscle tone, and of course, facial hair.

Despite its importance, the average testosterone level in men has fallen 25 percent in the past 20 years. In addition, 30 percent of men have testosterone levels that are too low. Without adequate testosterone, men become infertile, impotent, depressed, docile and weak—what a combo! In fact, men with low testosterone are 52.4 percent more likely to be obese, 50 percent more likely to develop diabetes, 42.4 percent more likely to have high blood pressure, and 40.4 percent more likely to have high cholesterol.

They also have little to no chance to grow significant facial hair. Before trying to Own Movember, it's critical to address low T.

The most common symptoms of low testosterone are:

-Very low or non-existent sex drive
-Erectile dysfunction
-Genital numbness
-Fatigue/low energy
-Low mood or depression
-Reduced muscle mass and weakness
-Increased body fat (specifically in the waist and man boob regions)
-Testicle shrinkage
-Facial and body hair loss

Any concerns you may have about your testosterone levels can be answered by a simple blood test. What constitutes low testosterone? It's really dependent on the individual, but most doctors will tell you that total testosterone levels below 350 nanograms per deciliter (ng/dL) are too low and need to be addressed. Your doctor will provide you with several options for effective treatment.

A man's testosterone level begins declining at age 30 and declines about 1 percent every year until he meets his demise. Optimizing your testosterone levels provide you with a whole host of health benefits and will give you the best chance to dramatically increase your beard coverage. It's a theme that will be revisited often in this book.

5
The Method Behind Our Madness

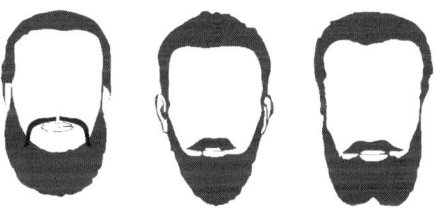

The quest to Own Movember is not an easy one; otherwise, everyone would own it! There are no shortcuts (well except for getting a facial hair transplant, which I discuss later) or miracle solutions. To transform your face you'll need to transform aspects of your life. Everyone will have a different starting point but the foundational theme remains the same.

There are two common approaches to increasing facial hair growth:

Inside-Out: You can attack the problem from the inside with diet and lifestyle changes, which will optimize your testosterone levels and turn your body into a hair-growing machine.

Outside-In: Attacking the issue from the outside-in, with various topical products and methods to stimulate and support additional growth from your facial hair follicles.

Both approaches have their plusses and minuses, so I naturally decided to combine them and fight my boy face on 2 fronts! Combining both approaches creates a powerful yet targeted method to rid yourself of boy face forever.

Part II: Inside-Out – Building Your Beard Growing Engine

Thurman Darby

6

Beard Food

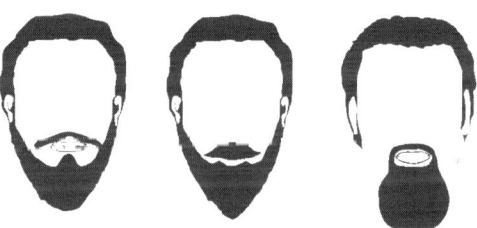

Your body is a factory, and if you want to it to perform at an optimal level, you need to fuel it with the right things. Diet plays a huge role in testosterone production and it's the source of vitamins and minerals needed to support facial hair growth. After moving out of my parents' house when I was 18, my diet had consisted of eating whatever was easy to get, cheap and tasted the best. It wasn't until my research for Own Movember that I learned by making some simple changes to my diet, I could dramatically enhance my beard-growing abilities.

Beer Bellies Need Not Apply

Some studies have found that just a 10 pound increase in abdominal fat can cut a man's testosterone in half. It's also been proven that with every 1 point increase in a man's body mass index (BMI), their testosterone level will decrease by a point.

If you're carrying a little excess weight in your midsection (most of us are), this is by far the number 1 thing you can do to positively impact your testosterone levels. This is because body fat converts a lot of testosterone into estrogen by releasing a conversion hormone called aromatase. Lucky for you, losing weight comes down to simple arithmetic: consume fewer calories than you burn and your body fat percentage will drop. You can tilt this equation in your favor by watching your calorie intake (not very fun) or by burning more calories than you do currently (a lot more fun). I actually increased my caloric intake during Own Movember because I was trying to build muscle, but I still managed to lose weight by becoming a lot more active. I joined volleyball, baseball, Ultimate Frisbee and trampoline basketball leagues which got me up and moving 3 nights a week.

There's a lot of great technology out there that will help you get an idea about how many calories you're burning daily. I also began a very efficient workout program—more on that in the next chapter. Although calorie counting is pretty lame, you will most likely need to change the type of foods you're currently consuming. Before Own Movember, my exposure to the 5 food groups was limited only by the toppings I could order on a pizza from my favorite pizza joint.

Own Movember Tip #5: Get your body fat percentage (especially in the abdominal area) as low as you can. Aim for a body fat percentage below 20 percent, with a range of 5 to 16 percent being optimal.

Here are some ways you can Own Movember with your diet:

Increase Your Protein Intake

Your hair is composed of protein, so naturally your hair loves a protein rich diet. Advice regarding the recommended amount of protein a man should consume daily is all over the map. The Dietary Reference Intake (DRI) states that 0.36 grams of protein per pound of body weight is enough, which is about 60 grams for a 170 pound man. That's pretty weak in my opinion and not nearly enough for our purposes. The actual amount a man should consume depends on factors like activity levels, age, muscle mass, physique goals and current state of health. My Own Movember diet consisted of 190 grams of protein per day, which equated to one gram consumed per pound of body weight. One gram per pound is also a common recommended amount for men working out several times a week and trying to gain muscle, which I was (more on the role of working out and muscle mass in the next chapter).

Own Movember Tip #6: Eat between 0.75-1.0g of protein per day per pound of body weight.

The benefits of a protein rich diet go beyond facial hair and muscle mass. Protein dulls hunger which helps prevent obesity. It also boosts testosterone. Like testosterone, your body does not store protein, so it's critical to ensure you are consuming enough of it every day.

The best sources of dietary protein are the following (calories per gram of protein):

1. Turkey Breast (1g protein/4.5 calories)
2. Chicken Breast (1g protein/4.5 calories)
3. Fish (Tuna, Salmon, Halibut, Snapper, Sole, Cod) (1g protein/4.5 calories)

4. Cheese (1g protein/4.7 calories)
5. Pork Chops (1g protein/5.2 calories)
6. Lean Beef (1g protein/5.3 calories)
7. Tofu (1g protein/7.4 calories)
8. Beans (not soybeans) (1g protein/10.4 calories)
9. Eggs (1g protein/12 calories)
10. Nuts (Peanuts, Almonds) (1g protein/15.8 calories)
11. Seeds (Pumpkin, Squash, Sunflower) (1g protein/15.8 calories)
10. Yogurt (1g protein/18 calories)
11. Milk (1g protein/18 calories)

In addition, here are some lesser known sources of protein:

Hemp Beans: No joke, these little beans pack a punch. They have a nice crunchy texture and a lot of flavor. They are an awesome source of omega 3 fatty acids and protein. I put them on my salads or just have them as a snack.

Shrimp: I'm a terrible cook, so I love how easy it is to add frozen shrimp to a meal. It can take anywhere from 4 to 15 minutes, depending on what kind of flavor profile you want. Shrimp are very low in fat and calories but chock full of protein and testosterone boosting vitamins like B12, D and the mineral selenium.

Green Peas: Again--I'm a terrible cook--so adding canned peas to a meal is really easy and you don't lose much nutritional benefit or taste versus getting them fresh. Peas are also incredibly easy on your wallet.

Peanut Butter: PB&J is still my favorite sandwich in the world and the PB part is full of protein and monounsaturated fats (a.k.a. the good fats).

Quinoa: God's gift to the protein-seeking vegan. Quinoa is a wonder grain that is high in protein, vitamins, and low in cholesterol. I'm not a huge fan but its meteoric rise in popularity over the last 10 years puts me in the minority.

Spirulina: What? I had never heard of this either. The blue-green vegetable plankton is alleged to have been the first photosynthetic life form ever created and is nothing short of a superfood. It's available in a lot of different forms at grocery and health food stores.

Eat Your (Cruciferous) Vegetables

Vegetables have been getting pushed on you since you were in diapers. You're well aware that they're great for your overall health but they're also great for your beard. Research has shown that consuming a diet rich in cruciferous vegetables (vegetables from the cabbage family) can help boost your testosterone.

Common cruciferous vegetables options include:

-Broccoli
-Cabbage
-Brussel Sprouts
-Collards
-Watercress (I had no idea what this was... it sounded like the name of a golf course)
-Kale (kale is so hot right now...kale)
-Kohlrabi (it looks like Sputnik... no joke!)
-Bok Choy

How many cruciferous vegetables should you consume per day? It's recommended that men get at least one serving of cruciferous vegetables per day. For Own Movember, I would try to at least double that.

Own Movember Tip #7: Eat at least 2 servings of cruciferous vegetables per day.

Fats Can Be Your Friend

For the past 40 years, health organizations have been preaching the importance of maintaining a low fat diet, yet during this low-fat revolution obesity rates have almost tripled. The truth is that we have been deceived! Not all fat is bad for you and in a lot of cases men aren't getting enough of it in their diets to maintain optimal health—that's right you heard me! Your body needs fat as it's a major energy source and helps you absorb certain vitamins and nutrients. More importantly, one of the most poorly understood nutritional facts is that testosterone is manufactured in the body from fatty acids! Yes, that's right; a diet deficient in certain types of fat will not only fail to increase your testosterone levels but will most likely cause it to fall significantly.

Own Movember Tip #8: Target 30% to 50% of your daily calories to come from healthy fats.

Here are the fats to be aware of to Own Movember (To ensure you can safely follow the guidelines provided, please consult with your doctor):

Fat Beard Fat: Saturated Fats

A previously condemned type of fat called saturated fat actually makes you more of a man—seriously! Saturated fat contains cholesterol, which is a precursor to testosterone. Saturated fats got a raw deal for decades when several flawed studies declared them nothing but artery clogging killers. It's only been in the past several years where health organizations have begun to change their position slightly. There's unfortunately still a ton of mixed information out there regarding saturated fat. It's pretty funny going back through time and seeing how often nutritional research studies contradict themselves because they're so poorly designed or their sample sizes are too low. One week a study concludes that eating pine needles decreases your risk of cancer by 15% and then the next week another study says that it increases your cancer risk by 40 percent and destroys your digestive tract.

Anyways, the studies that make the most sense to me conclude that a diet higher in saturated fat may raise your LDL or "bad" cholesterol levels but it may also raise your HDL or "good" cholesterol levels, which leaves your overall cholesterol profile in good shape.

OK, back to why you should care about saturated fat. Saturated fats are a proven testosterone creator. A notable study had 45 men initially given either a high fat/low fiber or a low fat/high fiber diet for 10 weeks and then after a washout period, they spent 10 weeks on the other diet. The high fat/low fiber period averaged 13% higher levels of total serum testosterone compared to the low fat/high fiber diet period. Similar studies have shown testosterone increases upwards of 30 percent.

The best dietary sources of saturated fats mostly come from animals and include:

-Fatty meats (beef, lamb, pork, chicken with skin)

-Cream
-Cheese
-Butter
-Ghee
-Lard
-Coconut oil
-Raw Chocolate
-Palm kernel oil
-Cacao butter

The common dietary guideline states that no more than 7 percent of your daily calories should come from saturated fat. Unless you have high blood pressure or high cholesterol, you should be able to safely increase that percentage a bit. During Own Movember, I averaged about 12 percent of my daily calories from saturated fat but I was also eating more calories per day. One gram of fat equals about nine calories and so I averaged about 33 grams of saturated fat per day.

Own Movember Tip #9: Saturated fats should make up between 7 to 12 percent of your daily calories.

Fat Beard Fat: Monounsaturated Fat

The "good" fat—eating a diet rich in monounsaturated fats (MUFAs) have been shown to dramatically improve your health in a number of ways. This includes increased testosterone levels, improved cognitive function, higher energy levels, lower risk of heart attack and stroke, reduced cholesterol levels, and weight loss.

MUFAs need to quickly become the number one source of fat in your diet. How much do you need? I targeted 30 to 40 percent of my calories per day, which on a 2,500 calorie diet equated to about 80 grams. This is incredibly easy to hit; a handful of macadamia nuts has over 80 grams of MUFAs!

Some great sources of monounsaturated fat include:

-Olives
-Olive oil
-Avocados
-Almonds
-Walnuts
-Flaxseeds
-Canola Oil

Fat Beard Fat: Omega-3 Polyunsaturated Fat

Another "good" fat is polyunsaturated fat. Polyunsaturated fats (PUFAs) can help reduce bad cholesterol levels in your blood which can lower your risk of heart disease and stroke. They also improve blood flow and circulation which not only help your beard growing but also your erection growing. The problem is that while PUFAs have positive effects on your overall health, most of them are known testosterone killers. A diet high in PUFAs has been shown to diminish testosterone production in men with one exception.

Polyunsaturated omega-3 fatty acids have been shown to positively impact the synthesis of testosterone. These compounds form the richest portion of fatty acids stored in testicular cells, and the testicles are the testosterone-producing glands in men. The other PUFAs (most notably omega-6's) shouldn't be avoided as they are essential but their consumption should be moderated. Mayonnaise and margarine are examples of food very high in omega-6 fatty acids.

Your best sources of omega-3 are:

-Flaxseeds
-Walnuts
-Sardines
-Salmon
-Fish oil
-Broccoli
-Radishes
-Other fresh fish

The Evil Fat: Avoid Trans-Fat

Trans-fats are toxic, highly processed, and basically unfit for human consumption. The moral here is to avoid these fats at all costs. Consuming trans-fats has been linked to heart disease and manages to simultaneously raise your bad cholesterol while lowering your good cholesterol. Trans-fat rarely occurs naturally as most of it is formed through an industrial process that adds hydrogen to vegetable oil, which causes the oil to become solid at room temperature. This partially hydrogenated oil is less likely to spoil, so foods made with it have a longer shelf life. Some restaurants use partially hydrogenated vegetable oil in their deep fryers because it doesn't have to be changed as often as do other oils.

Keep the Calories Coming

Your body needs a steady supply of calories to make testosterone, so regularly skipping meals or going for long stretches without eating can cause your testosterone levels to plummet. Research has demonstrated that low calorie diets are associated with lower testosterone levels. I think I skipped breakfast for over a decade and usually lunch too if things were busy at work. Skipping meals throws your body out of whack and shifts it into preservation mode since it doesn't know when its next meal will be.

Own Movember Tip #10: To keep your T levels elevated, ensure your body is getting calories at regular intervals. Never skip meals!

Getting Your Hair Growing Vitamins (and minerals) the Natural Way

Increasing facial hair growth isn't just about testosterone. It's critical to consume the necessary vitamins and minerals that promote hair growth. Here are the most hair-healthy vitamins to be aware of:

Biotin (Vitamin B7 or Vitamin H)
Beard Benefit: Improves your body's keratin infrastructure (a basic protein that makes up hair, skin and nails) and promotes hair and nail growth.
Best Food Sources: Whole-grain cereals, whole wheat bread, eggs, dairy products, nuts, salmon and chicken.

Vitamins B5 and B3
Beard Benefit: Circulation boosters.
Best Food Sources: Chicken, beef, fish, egg yolks, avocado, milk.

Folic Acid (Vitamin B9)
Beard Benefit: Necessary for the growth and repair of hair and promotes thicker hair.
Best Food Sources: Whole-grain breads, cereals, leafy green vegetables, peas, nuts.

Vitamin A
Beard Benefit: Encourages healthy hair follicles and sebum production (sebum keeps your follicles lubricated).
Best Food Sources: Carrots, broccoli, leafy green vegetables.

Vitamin C
Beard Benefit: Immune system booster which is essential to support hair growth.
Best Food Sources: Potatoes, green peppers, tomatoes and leafy green vegetables.

Vitamin E
Beard Benefit: Helps with your blood flow and promotes hair growth.
Best Food Sources: Beans, nuts and leafy vegetables.

Zinc
Beard Benefit: Zinc is important for the production of natural testosterone because it prevents testosterone from being converted into estrogen. Not only that, zinc helps your body produce healthier sperm and higher sperm counts.
Best Food Sources: Oysters (a natural aphrodisiac), liver, seafood, poultry, nuts and seeds.

Own Movember Tip #11: Ensure your diet is full of beard-friendly vitamins like biotin, B3, B5, B9, A, C, E, and zinc. If you can't get required amounts in your diet, use supplements.

Lay Off the Booze
     This one really hurt me. I come from a family of social drinkers—*very* social drinkers. I love having a few adult beverages on the weekend or after a long day of work. But as I researched

Own Movember, I was blown away at the negative effect that alcohol consumption has on a man's T levels. Alcohol fights your testosterone in almost every possible way.

Let me summarize its devastating effects:

1. Its products directly inhibit Leydig cells' production of testosterone.

2. Increases cortisol production (cortisol is the infamous stress hormone, and it blocks the production of testosterone).

3. Increases estrogen (alcohol slows down your body's ability to process estrogen, allowing it to build up in your blood stream and block the production of testosterone).

4. Decreases growth hormone production (heavy alcohol consumption disrupts your natural sleep rhythm).

Number 3 is the likely explanation why heavy drinkers begin to accumulate fat in the stomach (the sexy man-curve known as the beer belly) and pectoral region (a.k.a. man-boobs). A lot of the initial research I came across involved studying the effects of alcohol on rats (apparently scientists really like getting rats wasted). Anyways, those studies found that alcohol lowered testosterone in rats by 30 to 50 percent with even small amounts of booze having an effect.

Studies performed on men have come to similar but not quite as severe conclusions. One particular study measured men's T levels throughout a night of drinking. At the study participants' most intoxicated state, testosterone levels had dropped an average of

25% lower. In addition, when the subjects' blood alcohol levels were the highest, their testosterone levels were at their lowest.

Beer drinkers such as me get an added bonus. It turns out that hops (a key ingredient in beer) is one of the most powerful phytoestrogens (plant-based estrogens) in the world. Hops are so estrogenic that they are currently being studied as a treatment for hot flashes in menopausal women. If you want to optimize your testosterone levels, it's best to completely avoid alcohol but I know that will be an insane suggestion to some of you. Research has shown that even 2 drinks/day can lower your testosterone levels. I began swapping out beer for vodka when I did go out drinking, which I tried to limit to 1 or 2 nights a week at most.

Own Movember Tip #12: Try to drink in moderation 1 or 2 times a week.

No Soy for You?

I had always heard that consuming soy increased a man's estrogen levels so I tried to stay away from it as much as I could-- passing up a lot of delicious sushi and edamame beans in the process. However, research in recent years has largely disproven soy's alleged negative effects. Soy does not appear to have any significant effects on men's testosterone levels but it *does* appear to have cancer-fighting effects for men and women. Now that doesn't mean you should have Edamame beans and sushi for dinner every night, but the common belief that soy will turn you into a woman is incorrect i.e. consuming soy will not hold back your beard-growing efforts.

7

The Bigger Beard Workout

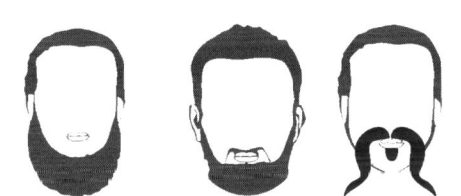

There are obviously a million reasons to work out and stay in shape. I won't lecture you on why it will make you feel better, look your best, and live longer. But what might surprise you is the crucial role working out plays in maximizing your beard growing potential. I'll admit it; I used to be a couch potato. It was a rarity not to see me in a sitting or horizontal position. I was hoping for a shortcut to beard growing riches. My initial attempts at increasing facial hair consisted of popping some supplements and applying a few lotions. It was as if the title of this book was going to be "The Coach Potato's Guide to a Bigger Beard." But of course there are no shortcuts in life or with beard growing.

Years ago, I was given a personal lesson in the power of working out from my very own flesh and blood. My younger brother and I come from the same gene pool and share a lot of the same physical characteristics, often being confused for identical twins when we were kids. Notably, we shared a complete lack of facial hair growing ability. But that changed drastically when he was about 21 (I was 22 at the time). That's when he began dedicating himself to personal fitness and transforming his body. Meanwhile, I remained a regular at McDonalds and on my couch. By the time of his 22nd birthday, we were no longer being mistaken for distant relatives let alone twins! He had grown himself a pretty decent looking beard with only a few patchy spots in less than 12 months! I was astonished. He also looked incredible physically. It was so blatantly obvious what caused such a dramatic physical change in his face yet I was blind to it. I regrettably continued my sedentary ways for many more years until my Own Movember transformation began.

It's been well established in this book that elevated androgen levels are the foundation of growing more facial hair. Without additional androgens circulating around in your blood stream, you're most likely not going to grow anything besides a beer gut. Nothing will naturally raise your testosterone to its optimal beard growing level like a properly designed work out program. I say properly designed because there are certain types of workouts and exercises that have dramatic body-transforming effects on men while other exercises will not produce any kind of meaningful change.

Getting the most of your workouts comes down simple arithmetic. Exercises that activate the most volume of muscle mass with the highest intensity will generate the most bang for your workout buck. This was a game-changing realization for me. Before Own Movember, when I actually did work out, I usually spent my time doing bicep curls and light running which did nothing but give me sore arms. After getting advice from my fitness-obsessed brother (who now looks like Mr. Universe), I learned that muscle isolating exercises like bicep curls should only be "the cherry on top" of your exercise program sundae. Those targeted, muscle isolating types of exercises don't become effective until you've spent significant time activating the giant muscle groups in your body. The best exercises to accomplish this are called compound exercises. Compound exercises are movements that use more than one muscle group and mobilize more than one joint. Exercises that target your largest muscle groups fire up your muscle building furnace and raise your testosterone levels. So what types of exercises am I talking about? Here's a rundown:

Squats – The King of Exercises

The squat is hands down the best compound exercise for men. It's the best exercise to gain muscle, build strength and boost your T levels. Squats are so effective because they activate and strengthen your largest, longest and most powerful muscles; these would be your glutes (the largest and most powerful), sartorius (the longest), and soleus muscles. Squats also strengthen your other big leg muscles like your hamstrings, calves, and quads.

What surprised me is that squats are actually a full body exercise. Your abs, lower back, obliques, shoulders, and arms are also actively involved. The best part is that all these different muscle groups are being worked at the same time and in the same motion.

Squats have a reputation for being bad for your knees but that's only if you use poor technique. I am far from an expert on weightlifting technique so I will leave that for the experts. If you don't have the assistance of a professional trainer, the best way to learn is by observing a professional. Youtube is full of great instructional videos that show you proper technique and tips to maximize your gains.

Deadlifts

The Deadlift is exactly what it sounds like—you're basically lifting a ton of dead weight off the ground. I believe it's the most important exercise next to the squat because it works all your big muscle groups with the heaviest weights possible.

Here is a rundown of the muscle groups worked when performing a proper deadlift:

-Your arms, forearms, and hands hold onto the barbell and make sure the bar stays in the right position and stays stable throughout the lift.
-Your shoulders and traps hold the weight and hold it stable.
-Your back and core help keep your entire body tight and stable to help keep your spine secure.
-Your posterior chain and legs to act as a lever to lift the weight.

The deadlift has the added bonus of not needing a spotter. However, your lower back is in a very vulnerable spot so start with lighter weights to perfect your technique.

Chin-ups – The Upper Body Squat

I love simple and chin ups are a very simple but extremely effective exercise that engages your entire upper body including your core. It's called the "Upper Body Squat" for a reason, and you'll feel chin ups powerful effects as soon as they're added to your workout routine. The motion is simple; you're essentially hanging from a horizontal bar and raising your chin to it, lifting your entire body weight.

Since heavy weights stimulate the most positive change in your body, you should try to add more weight to the exercise as soon as you can easily perform 10 repetitions. You can do this by purchasing a weight belt and attaching weights to it via a chain. When I first started seriously working out I actually placed weights in a backpack and wore it while I did the exercise.

Dips

Dips are another easy body resistance exercise that will efficiently stimulate your endocrine system to produce more testosterone and growth hormone. The motion involves suspending your body between 2 objects using your arms and "dipping" yourself down and up again. Dips are my favorite upper body exercise. I love doing them so much I recently purchased a $120 dip machine so I could do them properly at home. Similar to chin ups, once you can easily perform 10 repetitions you should add additional weight via a weight belt or backpack.

Military Presses

Another awesome upper body workout; the military press targets the deltoid muscles in the shoulders as well as the triceps but it also works the core and legs, which the lifter uses to help stabilize the weight. Military presses can be done with dumbbells or a barbell and in a standing or sitting position. Performing the exercise in a sitting position allows you to use heavier weight while standing brings your core and legs into play as stabilizers.

Own Movember Tip #13: Make squats, deadlifts, chin-ups, dips and military presses the foundation of your workout routine.

Workouts

I don't like spending hours at the gym; I like my workouts to be short but very efficient. Luckily for me, a man's body responds well to this time of workout. As I've previously mentioned, to maximize testosterone and growth hormone production, you should lift very heavy weights. Using weights that are about 80 percent of your single rep maximum should result in sets that are only 4 to 6 reps long. Research has shown that testosterone production is maximized at 3 sets per exercise with 1 minute rest periods in between. This is the workout framework that I used during my 12 month Own Movember program and what I continue to use now.

Own Movember Tip #14: Lift weights that are 80 percent of your single rep maximum. Do 3 sets of 4-6 reps resting 1 minute in between sets.

Post Workout

If you're doing all this hard work in the gym and not consuming adequate protein, it's almost counterproductive. Resistance training is so effective because it breaks down your muscles but you need to ensure that you're consuming enough protein so that it's available to repair and grow your muscles afterwards. The 60 minutes immediately after you workout is a time when your body is desperately trying to repair itself. This provides the most opportune time to infuse it with a protein boost. A study published in the American Journal of Clinical Nutrition pinpointed 20 grams as the best amount of postworkout protein to maximize muscle growth.

Own Movember Tip #15: To maximize your post workout gains, consume 20 grams of protein within 60 minutes of your workouts.

8

Testosterone Therapy

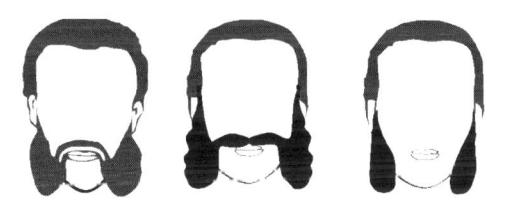

After reading the first 7 chapters of this book you may be thinking to yourself: "Why should I go through all the time, money and effort to do things that might raise my testosterone levels when I can just go the direct route?" I wondered the very same thing. There's a relatively newfound appreciation of the influence testosterone levels have over a man's quality of life, and with that men are increasingly turning to testosterone therapy.

Testosterone therapy is done under the close supervision of a doctor. This is important as too much testosterone or administering it incorrectly can have grave consequences and can not only result in severe health complications, but cause facial hair loss. Testosterone treatment may be done through injections, topical applications or oral ingestion. The third option is not recommended as it can often result in liver trouble. The testosterone can't be stored, so you may need to continue the regimen until you see facial hair growth. In some cases, testosterone therapy can take more than a year to provide results.

There are health risks associated with all types of testosterone therapy. The main risks are:

-Acne or oily skin
-Mild fluid retention
-Stimulation of prostate tissue, with perhaps some increased urination symptoms such as a decreased stream or frequency
-Breast enlargement
-Increased risk of blood clots
-Worsening of sleep apnea (a sleep disorder that results in frequent night time awakenings and daytime sleepiness)
-Decreased testicular size
-Increased aggression and mood swings

I've read of some gentlemen in the blogosphere who have had success with applying topical hydrocortisone to their face. Hydrocortisone is a steroid hormone. There is no official medical evidence to back up these claims and using hydrocortisone in that manner is very risky. Long-term use could have serious side effects, including blistering, skin damage, and hair growth on your forehead, back, arms, and legs (since its absorbed into your body). It could also result in lightening of the skin.

The side effects of testosterone therapy are dramatic enough to make it a very risky proposition for healthy men to take it just to supplement beard growth. Unless you do in fact have low testosterone, testosterone therapy is not something I would consider.

Part III: Outside-In – Targeting Your Efforts

Thurman Darby

9

Rogaine: What Works on Your Head Should Work on Your Face, Right?

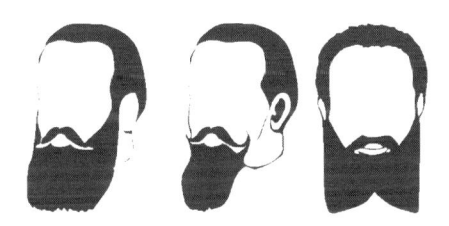

R ogaine is a topical solution available over-the-counter which has been approved in the US since the 1980's to treat male pattern baldness or "androgenic alopecia". Its active ingredient, monoxidil, was originally developed as an oral medication to treat high blood pressure. Rogaine has been a wildly successful product, generating billions in sales and saving the hairlines of countless men around the world.

Rogaine is advertised to "revitalize hair follicles and regrow hair" and despite a proven 30 year track record of results, its method of action isn't 100 percent clear. What *is* certain is that monoxidil is a vasodilator, which means it widens blood vessels and increases blood flow. The common hypothesis is that when it's applied to your scalp, monoxidil dilates the blood vessels in the area which increases blood flow to your hair follicles and rejuvenates them—makes sense right?

I had experience with Rogaine prior to my Own Movember journey. I had used it years earlier in an attempt to save the thinning hairline on my head. Reading testimonials of Rogaine will quickly tell you that it's very effective at preserving the hair that you currently have. In terms of actually regrowing new hair, it seems to be successful in doing so in about 40 to 70 percent of cases. I was lucky enough to be one of those successful cases, and after 8 months of consistent use, my hairline was significantly fuller. I was getting compliments on my hair for the first time in years. Naturally, I wondered whether Rogaine could work the same magic on my face. I soon became confident that it would.

Hair on your face is programmed by your genetics to respond in a specific way to the presence of androgens like testosterone. All men respond differently, but the response is almost always a positive one i.e. more androgen exposure, more facial hair. Mother Nature wasn't so kind to the hair on our heads; head hair is programmed differently than facial hair.

In some cases, hair head doesn't respond at all to increased androgen exposure. But for the unfortunate men like myself who suffer from Androgenic Alopecia, our head hair is genetically programmed to respond negatively to androgen exposure, specifically dihydrotestosterone (DHT). Consistent exposure to DHT over many years shrinks some of the follicles on our scalp and eventually puts them to sleep for eternity. In fact, the popular oral medication Propecia (generic name Finasteride) actually aims to reduce the levels of androgens that cause hair loss. The "Androgen

Paradox" is a term for this condition and it's important to know if you fall into it.

The increased androgen exposure which is so great for increasing facial hair could cause you to lose the hair on your head faster. It's not a deal breaker at all, and a lot of the tips and strategies in this book do not involve increasing androgen levels in your body. For me, the decision was easy. In my mind, I would've rather been a bald guy with a sweet beard a la Jason Statham or Randy Couture than a balding guy with weak facial hair. I was already losing the hair on my head and could always get a hair transplant if it began to bother me that much.

Rogaine needs to be used continuously or its positive effects will begin to reverse; the DHT attacking your head hair follicles will regain the upper hand. Your facial hair doesn't have the same problem. Anything you can do to stimulate the follicles on your face is pretty sustainable in the long term.

I did some research and found out that other men had tried Rogaine on their faces and had had success; so as part of my Own Movember strategy, I began applying a small amount of Rogaine foam to my cheeks and over my lip twice a day. I applied it in the morning and before I went to bed. Rogaine can irritate and dry out your skin, so it's OK to skip some applications as needed.

There are also side effects to be aware of (as there is with any medication). The side effects are described as occurring: "not very often" but if you do experience any stop using the product immediately. The most common side effects are skin itching, rash, and acne. I experienced some itching about two weeks in, but after taking a few days off I had no further issues. Other more serious side effects include blurred vision, chest pain, fast/irregular heartbeat, and dizziness. Very little of the active ingredient Monoxidil is actually absorbed into your system so if you have any side effects they will most likely occur on your skin but please do your own due diligence.

You can buy Rogaine without a prescription and it's widely available online at places like Amazon (is there anything they don't sell?) if you're embarrassed about buying it in person. A downside of Rogaine is cost; a box of Rogaine foam costs about $50 US (it's also available in a solution). A box would last me a month if I was just applying it to my face twice a day. Rogaine is off-patent so cheaper substitutes are available of its active ingredient monoxidil.

Own Movember Strategy #16: Apply a small amount of Rogaine twice a day to the areas of your face you want to stimulate hair growth.

10

Household Recipes

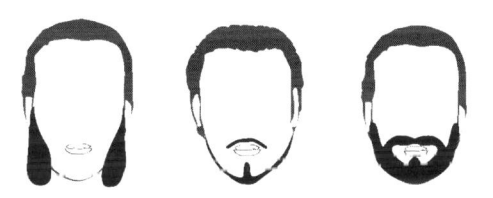

At one point, I was so desperate to grow some semblance of a real beard that I would have rubbed horse manure on my face if I thought it was going to help. Lucky for you, horse manure has not been proven to increase a man's facial hair growth (but it hasn't been unproven either). In my research, I discovered some creative items and concoctions that have had varying degrees of success for men around the world. Many of these items can be found in your average kitchen. I have tried a few of them and experienced generally positive results. These products are excellent alternatives if the cost or side effects of Rogaine aren't for you. If you notice any adverse reaction, discontinue application of these products immediately.

Eucalyptus

Eucalyptus oil comes from the eucalyptus tree found mainly in the bushlands of Australia. It's used for medicinal purposes like treating colds, sore throats and the flu. It's also a popular option to promote healthy hair growth due to its natural follicle-stimulating and scalp-cleansing qualities. Eucalyptus is definitely the real deal and I use it regularly on my face. The problem comes with how to use it. Eucalyptus oil will cause irritation to your face if applied to raw facial skin. To reduce irritation, mix it with something less irritating like olive oil and massage it into your face. If you have oily and acne-prone skin like me or detest the idea of using cooking oil as a skin product, look for eucalyptus-based products at your local drug store. I use a skin moisturizer and after shave with eucalyptus every morning.

Own Movember Strategy #17: Use face products with eucalyptus or rub a mix of eucalyptus oil and olive oil onto your face and leave on for 20 minutes daily.

Amla Oil and Mustard Leaves

Amla or the Indian gooseberry is said to be highly effective in increasing facial hair growth. It can be used alone or in combination with mustard leaves.

Option 1: Massage a little amla oil onto your face and leave it on for about 20 minutes; then rinse using cold water.

Option 2: Wash and grind a few mustard leaves into a paste and mix in a few drops of amla oil into this. Apply this paste to your face, leave it on for about 15 minutes and then rinse with cold water.

Do not use either option more than 4 times a week.

Own Movember Strategy #18: Massage amla oil or an amla oil/mustard leaf paste onto your face for 20 minutes 4 times a week.

Cinnamon Powder and Lime Juice

Mix one tablespoon of cinnamon powder with two tablespoons of fresh-squeezed lime juice. Blend the mixture thoroughly and apply the thin layer to you face. Leave it 25-30 minutes. Rinse your face with cool water and then wash with a gentle cleanser. Pat your face dry with a dry and clean towel, and apply moisturizer. Repeat this remedy twice a day, and stop once irritation occurs.

Own Movember Strategy #19: Mix cinnamon powder with 2 tablespoons of lime juice and put on your face for 25 minutes twice a day.

Cinnamon Bark and Lemon Juice

Powder a little cinnamon bark and mix one teaspoon of this with two teaspoons of lemon juice; apply this paste as a thin layer over the face the then rinse with cold water after 20 minutes. Use this solution about twice a week for best results.

Own Movember Strategy #20: Powder a little cinnamon bark and mix 1 teaspoon of this with 2 teaspoons of lemon juice and leave on your face for 20 minutes twice a week.

Coconut Oil

Coconut oil is fantastic for your hair and skin. It's used for everything from promoting soft and healthy hair to treating eczema. Apply a little onto a cotton ball and apply to your face, rinsing off with cool water after about 15 minutes.

Own Movember Strategy #21: Apply coconut oil to a cotton ball and apply to your face for 15 minutes.

Thurman Darby

11
Let's Get Surgical

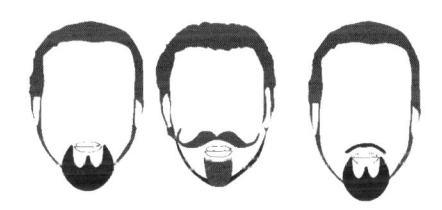

If you're not the patient type, the surgical route might be the best way to go. Just a few years ago, facial hair transplants were rare but are now being performed regularly by plastic surgeons around the world. The procedure takes hair follicles from an area on the patient's body (usually the head) and transplants them to areas on his face. It's a simple enough procedure that it's performed using only local anesthetic and is outpatient, meaning that you're home the same day. The most common complaint is minor irritation to the skin.

So what's the catch? Well the procedure costs anywhere between $5,000 and $15,000 USD depending on how much hair you're trying to move.

Side effects are described as minimal with the most common ones being:

Infection: There's a small risk of "folliculitis" or infection of the follicle. To prevent this, patients are given antibiotics for a week.

Swelling: Facial swelling that can last up to a week.

In-Grown Hairs: No explanation required here.

Patients are usually able to shave 10 to 14 days after the procedure. Facial hair transplants have a very high success rate and it was something I was going to pursue if I wasn't able to have success the natural way. If I get a scalp hair transplant in the coming years I may still opt for a "2 for 1" deal and fill in some of the patchier parts of my beard.

12
Growing, Coloring, Maintaining

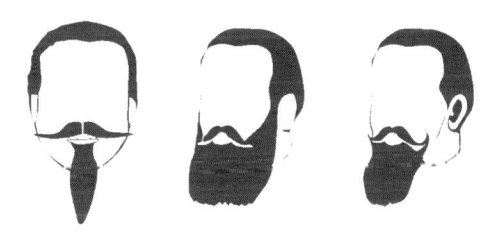

Men spend so much time focusing on their facial hair growing ability that they lose sight of the art and science of actually growing a beard. Knowing how to properly groom and shape your beard as it grows out makes a huge difference in how it looks. It takes at least 4 weeks to get any kind of fair sense about your beard growing ability,. That length of time gives your facial hair enough time to grow out, soften, and contour your face. It's also enough time for the hair to cover your patchy spots.

I was my biggest beard critic but soon realized I had never truly tried to grow one. After about a week of not shaving, I would become judgemental and self-conscious about my sparse collection of hairs. Depending on your dating and job situation, this might be difficult to overcome. As you begin to notice new facial hair growth, it will be important to try and take the leap to see exactly where you're at.

Own Movember Tip #22: It takes at least 4 weeks to get a true sense of your beard growing abilities.

So how can you make the growing out period less gross? This is where the all-important maintenance phase comes in. Facial hair maintenance is critical for all beard growers. First, buy yourself a decent beard trimmer. As you begin to grow out your facial hair and need to face the world, trimming is critical. Some of your hair will grow faster on certain parts of your face.

A few years ago, the hair on the very ends of my moustache grew at warp speed while the rest of it grew much slower. This created a very unattractive look for me if I did not intervene. As I began my Own Movember program and began to see progress, I would trim the sides of my mustache so the rest of it could catch up and even out.

Own Movember Tip #23: Buy a beard trimmer to help even out the hair growth on your face.

Another issue that I initially ran into was that of colour. I have blonde hair on my head, but when it came to my facial hair, it seemed to spout up in all colours of the rainbow. I would have groups of hair that would be jet black, while other hairs would be much lighter and almost invisible. A solution that really worked for me was purchasing the infamous "Just for Men" beard coloring gel. I initially laughed at the notion of using a product with corny commercials targeted at old men but after one application, all the invisible hairs came to life and it dramatically improved the look of my facial hair.

Own Movember Tip #24: To help give your facial hair a darker more uniform colour, use beard coloring gel.

Thurman Darby

13

Odds and Ends

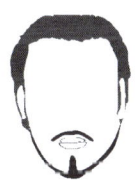

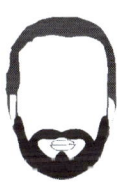

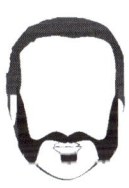

More Shaving, More Hair?

One of the most common questions I hear about facial hair is whether shaving more increases hair growth. There are all kinds of tales about hair getting darker and coarser after each time you shave it. Are the legends true? Well, not exactly.

Think of each hair on your face as a long thin tree branch; each tree branch is somewhat flexible when grown out. If you cut the branches down to a nub, they will be inflexible and appear thicker and stronger even though they are the exact same branches. Shaving your facial hair produces the exact same effect. After you shave, your facial hair begins growing back at the exact same speed and with the exact same thickness as it normally does—it just feels thicker initially because it's so short.

The real positive to shaving more if you're trying to grow more facial hair is that the act of shaving does stimulate your follicles—and stimulation often leads to growth—this applies to other areas of your body as well! Speaking of stimulation, another tactic I used is:

Send Your Follicles a Message with a Massage

Borrowing another treatment often given to balding jabronies like me; massaging the area in need creates blood flow to the hair follicles and stimulates growth. I definitely recommend this as it's easy, free and feels kind of nice. You can start with massaging your face 10-15 minutes twice a day—just make sure your hands are clean.

Own Movember Tip #25: Massage your face for 10-15 minutes twice a day.

Here are a few other tips that are effective but I didn't know where to put them in the book.

Give Your Boys Some Room to Operate

A man's testicles hang away from his body to be cooler. Heat can reduce sperm count and testosterone production. Try to wear looser fitting boxers—not briefs—and watch those long hot tub sessions!

Own Movember Tip # 26: Wear looser fitting underwear.

Shrink Your Penis but Grow Your Testosterone

We all know that cold water causes (temporary) shrinkage. But what isn't as known is the amazing effects it can have on your T levels. There's a famous story that the Soviet Weight Lifting team used to dip their testicles in ice water before competitions because it spiked their testosterone levels. I'm not suggesting you do that but hear me out. Keeping your boys cool helps them perform at an optimal level. Your testosterone levels are highest between 4am and 6am in the morning. Taking a cold shower at night before bed will naturally enhance your testosterone levels. I noticed it also helped me sleep.

Having another cold shower when you wake up will not only make you very alert (no morning coffee required!) but it will also give you a nice T level boost to start the day. As tough as I'm talking, cold showers are brutal. I've always been a guy who likes long, steamy, classic rock-filled showers. I was definitely looking for reasons for cold showers not to work for me but the problem is that they *do* work. I've noticed boosts in my energy levels, strength and mood since I began taking them.

My favorite time for a cold shower is actually after a workout when I'm hot and sweaty. The cold water seals in the heat and gives me a rush of endorphins. Try to stay in there for 10 minutes and keep the water as cold as possible. Also, try not to look down at your penis—it won't be pretty—but don't worry it should returns to its normal size.

Own Movember Tip #27: Take 1 cold shower per day that's at least 10 minutes long.

Final Words

So there you have it, that's everything I know about growing more facial hair and maximizing your facial-follicle growing abilities. By following a lot of the tips in this book, I was able to go from Movember chump to champ in 12 short months. I can't guarantee that you'll achieve the same results, but I *can* guarantee that you'll bring incredible amounts of positive change to your life in the pursuit of more facial hair.

I am currently in the process of developing a forum and website to post updates, new tips and testimonials from readers on their Own Movember journeys. In the meantime, feel free to send me an email at Thurman.Darby@Gmail.com if you'd like to share your thoughts on the book and what's working for you.

All the best,
-Thurman Darby

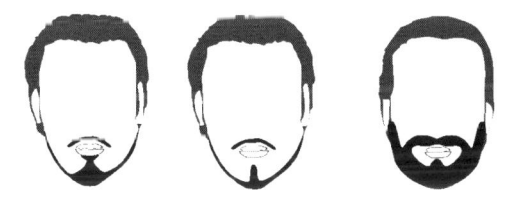

Thurman Darby

References

Brooks Robert C., Dixson, Barnaby J. (May 2013), The role of facial hair in women's perceptions of men's attractiveness, health, masculinity and parenting abilities. *Evolution and Human Behavior*. Volume 34, Issue 3, Pages 236-241.

Andersson AM, Jensen TK, Juul A, Petersen JH, Jørgensen T, Skakkebaek NE. Secular decline in male testosterone and sex hormone binding globulin serum levels in Danish population surveys. *J Clin Endocrinol Metab.* 2007 Dec;92(12):4696-705. Epub 2007 Sep 25.

Thomas G. Travison, Andre B. Araujo, Amy B. O'Donnell, Varant Kupelian, and John B. McKinlay. A Population-Level Decline in Serum Testosterone Levels in American Men. *The Journal of Clinical Endocrinology & Metabolism* 2007 92:1 , 196-202.

Sierksma A, Sarkola T, Eriksson CJ, van der Gaag MS, Grobbee DE, Hendriks HF. Effect of moderate alcohol consumption on plasma dehydroepiandrosterone sulfate, testosterone, and estradiol levels in middle-aged men and postmenopausal women: a diet-controlled intervention study. Alcohol Clin Exp Res. 2004 May;28(5):780-5.

Printed in Great Britain
by Amazon